Best Foot Forward

Moving on From Anxiety

Printed and bound in England by www.printondemand-worldwide.com

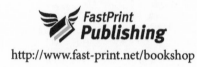

http://www.fast-print.net/bookshop

Best Foot Forward

ISBN 978-178456-538-1

First published 2018 by
FASTPRINT PUBLISHING
Peterborough, England.

Best Foot Forward

Moving on From Anxiety

Lyn Halvorsen

And the night shall be filled with music,

And the cares, that infest the day,

Shall fold their tents like the Arabs,

And as silently steal away.

From 'The Day is Done'

Henry Wadsworth Longfellow

Contents

Contents

Introduction

Hello and thank you for finding this book. Whatever happens to any of us in life, we all need a friend at times, even if they just turn up and buy the coffee. Simple actions help because it means someone is giving time to you, which is a gift. I hope you will find some words here to comfort you, help you, or at least cheer you up for a while; that would be my gift to you.

The following pages contain some words and observations about anxiety. There are many books written about the subject, as there are many of us who suffer from it. In the following pages I want to write about a few ways of coping with anxiety that you may find helpful. I'm not here to offer fancy solutions or amazing new remedies (of course if I had them I would), and I am not a practising medical person. My credentials, if you are interested are as follows:

I was a nurse for many years so there is not much that shocks me.

I am a wife, mother and grandmother (of nine) so I know a bit about the workings of family life.

I am a writer and it is important to me to write about the positive and peaceful side of life.

I believe in love and kindness with a bit of humour thrown in.

Some of my writing here is based on anxiety and how it has affected me and real people that I know or have known. This is not because I am being a bit indulgent, it is more to illustrate the various guises anxiety can take and to show you what might work to help. Personally, I feel it helps when I read about other people's experiences, so maybe reading about mine will help you.

Here's the thing: I listen to and follow so much advice from my various favourite lifestyle gurus - you know, the ones who speak calmly at us through our headphones and lead us to believe that we only have to meditate every day, visualise our dreams and stay in a good calm place to have the world sussed out, that I find myself questioning why some days I don't feel better than I do. I have always been one to worry a bit about things although I have perfected the art of putting on a brave face, and there are still days when I wake up feeling quite fearful.

On days such as these, I bring out the essential oil burners, the 'spiritual fitness' (soothing) music goes on and I read my favourite books for inspiration and reassurance. I may even consume the healthiest breakfast I can manage, overflowing with the juiciest blueberries and sprinkled with turmeric powder. Superfoods make me feel better. Often I head for the woods to commune with nature. Being outside always helps, and worries and cares never seem so overpowering. So then I face the day with renewed optimism. Probably for ten minutes. Then I remember I have to send a recorded voice message to a client, which I rehearse to be sure it sounds professional. I send said message. So why do I sound like the Queen on a bad day? (I'm not being disrespectful here – I admire the Queen.) Where has my normal voice escaped to? Why does nervousness, when it takes over, alter all our regular actions and allow them to be feeble or peculiar, or even, frankly, embarrassing? (Anyone who has experienced the jerky/shaky head movements can probably sympathise with me here.) Okay. Time for a reality check, or actually, maybe an un-reality check, for what is real and what is imagined here? I realise I am looking too far ahead, visualising all the things that could go wrong but probably won't. I have lost my perspective and even my gratitude. Gratitude for the day I have been given, and which I am now wasting with negative thinking.

One thing I am now teaching myself is to be present. Be where I am and not where my anxiety wants to take me. I remind myself that an anxious mind is actually a strong mind, as anyone who has tried to rationalise themselves out of being anxious will tell you. Anxiety exists in all of us at times - we wouldn't be human if we didn't experience it, and of course, it is primarily there to keep us out of danger and to strengthen us if we harness it in the right way. But of course, being on high alert all the time is not good for us, and can drain us of our vital energy. So I remind myself I can be bigger than the anxiety: stronger and more resilient. I won't fight anxious thoughts but tell myself I have no need for them today. I am comfortable and safe and I am okay. If I accept I am sometimes anxious it doesn't have such a grip on me and it loses energy and power.

We can read all the information we can get our hands on.

Some days it helps and we find a nugget of wisdom that really shines like a beacon and has a profound effect; other days not so much. Maybe those are the days we should watch a 'feel-good' film or eat some chocolate (okay, it's organic). But at least there is a lot of help out there if we embrace it. And there is one thing I urge you to think about if you suffer from anxiety: you are not alone. The 'self-help' industry is huge. There are gurus everywhere - we could probably each have our own personal one there are so many - so remember, many of us are searching for help and many of us want to use our own experiences to help others. There is always room for a new way of looking at things, and for new ideas. Techniques we laughed at yesterday could be the most beneficial and accepted way of helping us tomorrow.

Talking about laughter, humour is the best way for me to deal with anxious situations. It's not easy to be funny or feel amused on demand but trying to look on the funny side helps. I always think the saying we should love ourselves sounds particularly cheesy, but if we do, then we can look upon a bit of laughter as a good way of healing, and one that stops us beating ourselves up when we feel low. Laughter scares away depression and activates happy feelings, and we as humans are wired to respond positively to laughter and smiles. So there we can tell ourselves that we are at least helping others if we wear a smile.

So next time I hear myself sounding like Her Majesty I will smile and make the most of it. By doing that I will probably relax and return to being my normal self too!

Before we start, I add this: it's not just a legal disclaimer – I care enough about you to say that if you are feeling really terrible and just cannot find a way out, then please find a doctor you can trust to help you through; sometimes self-help isn't enough on its own and there is absolutely no reason to put off seeking medical treatment when you need it.

This book is really a collection of my thoughts and suggestions for coping with anxiety. There is the odd bit of advice here and there, but mainly I have given observations. Any use of information in this book is at your (the reader's) discretion and is not intended to replace medical advice.

We are all different and unique and look for our own ways to cope with this crazy life. I hope you open the book and find some words that help you take a happy and contented path.

This book has been adapted from my blog
www.notesfromdovelane.com

There are many ways you can seek help if you need it and there is more information at the end of the book for this.

What is Anxiety?

Anxiety takes many forms and can shape your thought processes and decisions. Characterised by an unpleasant state of inner turmoil, it is thought to be related to the biological fight or flight response to feeling threatened. It can become a problem if it is accompanied by panic attacks or anxiety about things which are part of everyday life. Anxiety is not the same as fear, which is a response to a real or perceived immediate threat; it is the expectation of a future threat.

Anxiety isn't rational. It's not just an amplified version of what is worrying you. It's more than that. Sometimes you don't know what sets it off. Some days you can cope with life and others you just don't want to know. A lot of people think anxiety is nothing more than a similar feeling you get before giving a presentation at work or an actor having first-night nerves; it may be a bit like that at times, but often it's more long-lasting and doesn't decrease as it would when events like the above are over. Some of the symptoms are palpitations, wanting to escape from your surroundings, fear you may lose control of thoughts or actions, racing heart, nausea, insomnia and nervousness, muscular tension, fatigue and restlessness. The list can be almost endless.

Anxiety can strike anyone and people from all walks of life. It doesn't really matter what your circumstances are, what background you come from, whether you are in a happy relationship or alone, hold down a high-powered job or are unemployed, well-off or hard up. It can creep up on anyone and sometimes it is just unexplained.

Fear of Loss

Most of our anxiety comes from the fear of losing something or someone that we perceive as being very important to us. This may include a loved one, our own health, our job, perhaps even our wealth. Sometimes it may be seemingly minor things like losing face with our peers.

Loss of control can affect us deeply. If we let go of the reins what will happen? How will we appear to others and what will the effects of change mean to us? These are questions we often ask ourselves and can keep us tossing and turning at night.

Anxiety and Behaviour

There are some times in life when we are severely affected by life-changing events, such as loss of a loved one, divorce, financial disaster or major ill-health and of course this will deeply affect and alter our equilibrium. Deep stress, sadness and anxiety will be a major factor here and will naturally command the sympathy and love of those around us, which will hopefully help us to heal or at least adjust or accept. But the anxiety that we find affecting us in ways that are harder for us or others to understand can be the type that is seen or labelled as irrational. We ask ourselves why we are feeling this way when life is seemingly good and we have no real reason to feel such turmoil.

Anxiety is an emotion that affects us negatively and affects our behaviours in so many ways and can make everyday life stressful. Sometimes, rather than go through a situation that has made us anxious in the past, we would rather side-step it or avoid it altogether. By affecting our mood it can affect our relationships and our well-being. Anxiety is tiring. All those unsettling thoughts and unexplained worry drain your energy and that in turn makes you feel worse.

Anxiety can cause both physical and emotional distress, and many people experience anxiety from time to time; when times are challenging it can make symptoms worse. In a way, it may help to remind yourself that it is part of a very human experience from which no one is immune. In the following pages I will go through the various causes and triggers of anxiety and hope to help you find some answers to why you feel as you do, and ways to move forward.

This is a time for self-compassion and speaking kindly to yourself. Remember – 'this too will pass'. When you find a way through, and come out the other side, you will feel great accomplishment and be well-armed for the future.

Causes of Anxiety

Many things trigger anxiety. What makes me anxious may not seem a worry to you and vice versa.

There is a difference between a trigger of anxiety and a cause of anxiety. For example, something that you have experienced earlier in your life has caused the anxiety you suffer from today, whilst triggers are issues that 'stir up' your anxiety. Not everyone who suffers with anxious feelings experience them every day. Some people may have long spells where they feel okay about life. Others may have prolonged spells where they feel their anxiety is particularly bad. If triggers for anxiety occur frequently then the anxiety may become hard to manage.

Causes from the past

This is not a time to apportion blame, but often our propensity towards anxiety can be passed down to us from family members. If we witnessed severe reactions to everyday events as well as traumas in our childhood, and grew up thinking this was normal, it is no surprise that we may follow a similar pattern of behaviour should similar circumstances present themselves. Your sub-conscious mind will produce the same negative emotional response.

When did we start to get anxious? Could it have been when we were very small and expected to behave well? Did we feel shy or awkward? Were we praised and encouraged enough or were we made to feel bad if we underachieved? Could it have arisen from schooldays? Were we expected to perform; to pass exams? Were we told there would be dire consequences if we didn't do well? Did we feel pressured to eat all our food or teased about our body shape or size? Often this can lead to problems with eating in later life. Maybe we grew up thinking we always had to please people.

Did you have a severe trauma in your past which you have buried deep in the recesses of your mind? The wound may have healed over, but the scar, though perhaps faded, will forever remain. I am not urging you to reopen old wounds but to take a look at what could be the cause of your anxiety and acknowledge it. Once you do that, with help and understanding, you can find ways of dealing with bad memories from the past.

Everyday life can be a cause of anxiety. We are bombarded with news from all aspects of the media, which is predominantly negative. We see terrible acts of violence and terrorism, cruelty and suffering unfold graphically before our very eyes. How can we bear to see such fear and sadness? We may ask ourselves what is happening to our world and witnessing these events may cause us to lose perspective. We may perceive the world as a hostile and an unfriendly place to be.

We may be affected by our environment. Our surroundings appear to be much more affected by climate change, pollution, noise, and negative energies. Sometimes we do not always visibly see what is causing our unrest.

Films and video games are available to watch on our screens and it is possible to be distanced from reality.

Diet

It is easy to assume that our diet is nutritious. Even when we think we eat a balanced diet there is always room for improvement. With the busy lives most of us lead, it is easy to grab whatever food is going or eat fast food and 'takeaways'. Highly processed foods not only are devoid of nutrients but can be positively harmful to our mood and well-being. The main 'baddies' which we would all do well to avoid are: processed foods, all sugars, fried foods, cured meats, sodas, excess caffeine and alcohol. These foods can create inflammation in our bodies by harming our digestion. Poor diet will contribute to poor gut health which could lead to 'leaky gut' and IBS symptoms. If we do not absorb our nutrients as nature intended, our bodies can be more prone to disease and depression.

Many scientists now believe that the key to our well-being

is related to our gut health. Our gut health is related to our diet. In a healthy gut, seventy percent of our serotonin is produced by the healthy microbes that live in the stomach. Serotonin is one of the most important chemicals in our brain for promoting the feeling of well-being. How often do we hear people say: 'My gut feeling was to do this or not to do that'? Our feelings and lifestyle affects our gut in many ways and, in reverse, our gut health affects our thinking quite dramatically. When we are anxious we get 'butterflies in our tummy' and often a churning feeling, proving that there is a direct connection with our gut and our brain. So a quieter mind will help our gut feel more settled. There are many studies which show how beneficial pre- and probiotics can be in aiding our digestion by supplementing our gut flora or bacteria, which in turn may help us feel calmer overall.

Whatever diet you follow, be it vegetarian, vegan, paleo or 'hunter gatherer' for example, try and make it as wholesome as you can. Just because a diet has a label doesn't mean it is always healthy. It helps to do your research to find out what diet suits your body-type best and to ensure your food comes from the best source you can find. At the same time, don't get too hung up about your diet either. Do your best to eat well but if you have a few lapses and indulge in a cake or two now and again don't beat yourself up. If you enjoyed it, it probably did you good in a 'feel-good' way!

Avoid any foods that trigger your anxiety and cause headaches, like cheese or yeast extract, for example. Acid-producing food and drinks can make you jittery, i.e. processed meats and sodas, whilst alkaline foods can be more calming, i.e. vegetables and most fruits, beans and lentils. Sometimes when you eat certain foods you may notice a pattern emerging –i.e. tiredness, mental fogginess or bloating, and this may indicate these foods do not suit you and may be best avoided.

I do not feel that one diet suits everyone, and you may have certain ethical reasons for wanting to follow a certain diet, or you may prefer to avoid dairy/wheat, etc. All I suggest is that you eat good and nutritious food which is as unadulterated as possible. Other possible choices to consider for boosting your health are juicing and, of course, drinking enough water. In these days of intensive farming and modern agriculture, some foods may not contain as many nutrients as they once did and therefore going for organic and bio-dynamically produced foods would be better. However, this may not always be financially sustainable, and so you might want to consider a multi-vitamin and mineral supplement to top up your diet. I feel this has benefited my own personal health but it is very much personal choice. If you do decide to supplement your diet it is worth asking for advice from a good nutritionist or naturopath.

'Let food be thy medicine and medicine be thy food.'
Hippocrates

Exercise

Exercise can really help to alleviate stress and anxiety. The problem can be that when we feel down or anxious we lose motivation to do anything, let alone go out and take exercise. But take small steps if you really feel lethargic. Make the effort to go out and walk around the block and you will soon feel uplifted. Nature has a way of working magic! Who can fail to be cheered up by the sight and sound of a merry robin singing his heart out in the tree above their head, or the beauty of the sun bursting through the clouds on a grey day? If you can get used to taking a daily walk you can increase your distances and improve your fitness. Walking, especially at a brisk pace, can really improve your physical and mental health. Of course, you may be used to exercise and have just got a bit out of practice and if that is the case try and resume those sports/hobbies (if you enjoy them!). Sometimes it's good to walk with a friend and chat as you go. Leave your worries behind you and concentrate only on what is around you and the power of nature. What works for me is putting on the headphones and listening to some inspiring music or listening to an audio of one of my favourite motivational speakers, whilst walking in the woods behind my house. Overall, exercise is one of the most effective ways of improving your mental health. Regular exercise can have a profoundly positive impact on depression, anxiety and stress. It will also help you sleep better and will boost your overall mood.

The Importance of Sleep

Good quality sleep is so important. Ideally we should get eight hours a night. With families to look after and demanding jobs or even a thriving social life, we often do not get that peaceful night's sleep that we should. Sleep plays a big role in your physical health and mental health. For example, sleep is involved in healing and repairing your body and supporting good brain function. In children and teenagers, sleep also helps support growth and development so perhaps we shouldn't be too hard on our teenagers when we have trouble getting them out of bed! Lack of sleep can impact on us in many ways and even harm over time; deficiency can raise your risk of some chronic health conditions such as diabetes and heart disease, and can also affect how well you think, react, work, learn and get along with others. It can affect our safety too; if we are tired when performing important tasks such as driving or operating machinery we can be prone to accidents. Children who suffer from lack of sleep may struggle with school work and examinations.

Sleep helps your brain work properly. While you are sleeping, your brain is preparing for the next day; it is forming new pathways to help you learn and take in information. It may be that sleep deficiency alters activity in some parts of the brain, so if you are sleep deficient you may have trouble making decisions or controlling your emotions and behaviour. It will also play a part in anxiety and depression.

Sleep is important in regulating the hormones in your body such as insulin, which controls your blood sugar, and important growth hormones in children. Another interesting point is that lack of sleep makes you hungry, so if you battle with your weight and controlling your eating it may be worth thinking about a few early nights!

Melatonin and sleep
The pattern of waking up naturally when it is light and sleeping at night when it is dark is a natural part of human life. A key factor in how we sleep is regulated by exposure to light or darkness. You may say this is obvious, but in modern

times we do not really sleep in the way our ancestors did or indeed as animals do. Melatonin is a natural and beneficial hormone produced by the pineal gland in your brain. During the day this gland is inactive. When the sun goes down and darkness occurs, the pineal gland starts to function and releases melatonin. This has the effect of naturally slowing the body down and preparing us for sleep. When we sleep, melatonin levels stay elevated in the body and then fall again with the light of the new day. So we see that light affects how much melatonin the body produces. During the shorter days of winter, your body may produce melatonin either earlier or later in the day than usual and this change can have an effect on mood, often called seasonal affective disorder (SAD). It is good to make sure your curtains are drawn at night and the bedroom is dark; all appliances should be switched off and try not to have a television in the room! Leave your mobile out of immediate range too! (It can be done!) All electronic devices can interfere with your sleep. One thing I try and do (and often find it hard to stick to) is to have a 'wind-down' spell after 8pm. This means staying away from the computer and leaving unfinished work until the next day. Most emails can wait until the morning! Also, I try to avoid listening to late-night news so that I don't go to bed feeling troubled.

In the dark night hours, there is nothing much worse than lying awake tossing and turning. Every minor problem and worry about tomorrow becomes magnified and before you know it you have a whole list of possible bad scenarios bubbling up in your mind. The best thing to do in this situation is to get up. Instead of staying in bed worrying about how many hours of sleep you will be missing and fearing you will be a wreck the next day, go and make a warm drink and try and clear your mind with some calm thoughts. Do something else for thirty minutes until you feel really tired. Just be sure it's not something too stimulating or involving bright light.

When lying in bed, try relaxing all the muscles in your body from head to toe. This is called Progressive Muscle Relaxation and is a good way of winding down when you get into bed at night. Once you are laying quietly, work through your muscle groups from head to toe. Start with your face: lift your eyebrows and wrinkle the forehead, then close your eyes tight before opening them and relaxing. Tense your lips, cheeks and jaw muscles by grimacing, then feel the serenity come over you as you relax all your facial muscles. Work down through the body, tensing and then relaxing the shoulders and arms, the chest and abdomen, (breathing deeply and exhaling as you relax), the back muscles, hips and buttocks, and lastly, the legs and feet. After you have systematically tightened and relaxed all the muscle groups in your body, you should feel more relaxed and calm. You may even fall asleep half-way through!

Relaxation CDs

I love to listen to soothing music at night. It's great for helping you drift off. I recommend some CDs at the back of this book.

Sleep is very important in helping put away the thoughts from yesterday; with good restful sleep the brain can organise and sort the good thoughts from the bad and do away with 'mind chatter' so you can awake refreshed and ready to face a new day with new mental awareness. During the day, and often the evening too, especially during the winter, I have a Himalayan salt lamp plugged in. I have read various reports about their possible health benefits, such as cleansing the air, helping to reduce allergies, increasing energy levels, helping with sleep, treating seasonal affective disorder, and producing an environmentally friendly light source. Whatever their benefits, I do know they certainly lighten up any room with their friendly warm glow and seem to freshen the air too. You can place them on a desk, in your living room, next to the bed or anywhere you choose.

When you are awake at night and feel the darkness closing in, remember that everything will feel better in the morning. Okay, not everything perhaps, especially if you have any ongoing troubles, but you will be able to put things more into perspective when you are up and about, have opened the curtains, and chased away the night. And if you do lie awake worrying, remember also that there is nothing at all you can do about anything in the night-time hours, so you may as well get to sleep and think about it again another time!

'As the sun sets, fold away your cares of the day and leave them outside your door. Then, wait to glimpse the moon and stars and know the Universe is wiser than we can ever be.'

Triggers of Anxiety

There are several obvious understandable natural triggers for anxiety: a stressful job, for example. Living with disease can create anxiety, whether it is your disease or someone close to you. Trouble with relationships or your social life is another common trigger.

Stress in the Workplace

Whether you are a business owner, self-employed or an employee, anxiety can be caused by work as well as other personal issues and problems. Some common causes of stress at work include excessively high workloads or unrealistic deadlines which can make you feel rushed, under pressure and overwhelmed. There are many compliance issues these days which, although they may be necessary, can be very time-consuming and worrisome. As mentioned before, anxiety often involves worrying about the future and this can often become apparent when thinking about future career prospects. Your job may be high-powered and exacting but sometimes the opposite can be a problem, i.e. feeling undervalued and feeling you are not living up to your potential. Perhaps interactions with colleagues may cause you worry, or even a stressful journey every day just to get to work. High levels of anxiety at work are a well-known cause of poor performance and absenteeism and can manifest physically with symptoms such as headaches, back pain and even panic attacks. Often anxiety is very subjective and it is important to talk to someone about your concerns. Do you have a supervisor or a colleague you could talk to? Sharing the problem with a partner or friend may help too. Perhaps you could make some notes for a few weeks to identify which situations seem to be cropping up the most, and then you can work out the best way to respond to them. Excess anxiety in the workplace can permeate through to your family and loved ones and even spoil your valuable leisure time so you owe it to yourself and those around you to find a way to manage your anxiety. Would you even consider changing your job if you felt you were not fulfilling your potential or being appreciated? Sometimes you need to meet some searching questions about your lifestyle head-on. A radical change may be far more beneficial than you think, even though the idea may be very challenging.

Living with Illness

Sadly, some of us or someone we love may be diagnosed with an illness which can be devastating, possibly life-threatening and/or debilitating. This will arouse so many emotions and fears that one can feel shaken to the very core. Our deepest anxieties are unleashed, and fears for our future and the future of those we love are uppermost in our minds. If we allow these deep fears to dominate our thinking we will fuel our fears even more, whereas if we take up a more proactive and optimistic way of thinking we can become more positive and look into ways of improving our situations. Even small changes will help us to think more about a better way forward for either ourselves or those we love. Our minds and thoughts are very powerful and if we can use them to improve our outlook it is surprising how miracles can occur.

Worry about Finances

Nearly all of us, whoever we are, worry about our finances. It is not confined to the less wealthy amongst us. Even billionaires worry about how to manage their money! When our financial situation gives us serious cause for concern for whatever reason, we can feel our anxiety levels rocket. Our greatest dread can be eviction, not being able to provide for our families, loss of face amongst our peers, shame...the list goes on and on. We fear we cannot survive, which is our basest fear. Of course, I do not know what you may be facing at the moment but, I promise you there is always a way out, even if you cannot see it yet. This will pass eventually. Do not be afraid to ask for help; you will find there is more out there than you think and, most people are inherently kind when it comes down to it. Life may change dramatically but don't let pride and ego get in the way of seeking help and starting again.

Downsizing

This is something which I have experienced personally, and was an unexpected and unwelcome change. My husband and I downsized several years ago for various reasons. For a long time, this was nothing short of horrendous. We left a big house in the country which we loved and ended up renting different houses until our circumstances changed and we found a house we were happy with. Each time we moved, we had to sift through our belongings and give various items away. We lugged bits and pieces to and from storage units until we were left with…not very much. But we learned a hard lesson. When we finally sat down in the latest home and put our feet up we realised we didn't need all the trappings we had been clinging on to for so long and life actually became more orderly. We had found our way through the chaos. And as long as I could keep hold of my very precious and personal keepsakes, I realised I didn't need a lot else. (By the way, there is not much I don't know about the stresses and strains of moving, but maybe I will save that for my next book…)

The only thing I will add is that we now find ourselves settled and in a state of gratitude (most of the time). For us, we were able to get back on our feet, but if you find yourself having to move house or losing your house for whatever reason, it can be a devastating blow and I am well aware that for some people even homelessness or displacement may be the outcome. Here it would be hard not to be anxious and feel deep despair, but even in the most distressing of situations if we cling on to hope and reach out to those who can help us we can find a way through.

For a while after we had downsized I felt as though the axis of my world had shifted. I even felt people were treating me differently. So many times we mix with people who seem to have it all. We may ask ourselves why we can't be like them. They appear as though they don't have a care in the world. Often I have formed an opinion of someone before I have had a chance to get to know them. I have made an assumption that their life is bordering on perfect, only to find out later on that they have worries and problems similar to mine. It's a good thing to remember that most people, whoever they are, may be fighting battles within themselves that we know nothing about. When we were going through rather traumatic times we carried on as best we could and most people we knew didn't really realise how bad we were feeling. It seems to be what we do: put on a brave face and carry on. Perhaps we feel we are giving in if we crumble. We are anxious to show we are **not** anxious!

Self-Image
We have multi-billion-pound industries devoted to telling us how we should look and present ourselves to the world. This

begins when we are young children and is promoted on a world-wide and daily basis and is a never-ceasing bombardment. This can affect people in all social and economic groups. Even the most self-assured amongst us may think twice before we go out if we are not feeling 'up to the mark'. If we don't feel we 'fit in' we become uncomfortable and try and be like everyone else. Society wants us to conform even though deep down this may not suit us. It is hard at times to remind ourselves that our lives are not dependent on what others think. Even when people are well-meaning, they are often taken up with their own lives and appearances and are not in the least worried about how we appear to them; often all the angst we go through when worrying how others see us is just a waste of energy. If you enjoy being a follower of fashion or the latest trends then that's great, but if not, just be happy with who you are. And remember, if you were a good and kind friend to someone, they will remember the kind actions you showed them rather than what you were wearing!

Relationships

For most of us, our deepest desires include having good and long-lasting relationships. Partners, children, friends and acquaintances are the foundations of our own personal world. Love is the most powerful emotion possible, and when you start to experience anxiety over that love, it can profoundly affect the way you view a relationship and even everything around you. If you sense a relationship is coming to an end for whatever reason, the fear of loss can be overwhelming, as can the fear of being alone.

So many things can cause anxiety in relationships, some very serious and others less so, and the anxiety levels can vary depending on the cause. Whatever the cause though, if it is making you anxious, it will be something you want to make better or move on from. Abusive relationships can cause anxiety for reasons that are entirely different from those that arise from bringing up children, for instance. Other causes of worry are loss of trust, perhaps about uncertainty for the future in a relationship, or infidelity, disagreeing over family issues, negative thinking in a partner, or a 'staleness' in a relationship.

Putting a stop to relationship anxiety takes time and patience. Relationships can be very complicated and often issues may have been smouldering away for some time. It takes courage to bring out things which have been covered up to avoid upset and change. But until we communicate our thoughts, who can really know what has been bothering us all this time? The person you have an issue with may be at a loss to know what is upsetting you until you talk about it.

There are two things to ask yourself long before you can expect to put things right or move on. The first is whether you want to remain in a relationship, and the second (which applies if you have a relationship problem with a partner) is: are you willing to change even without your partner changing?

One thing to remember is that you can't change other people, you can only change yourself. There are questions only you can ask yourself and affirmations you can follow. Do you remember why you married or set up home with your partner in the first place? Can you re-ignite the magic and joy you felt when you were first together? Do you still admire their qualities - the uniqueness and quirkiness that attracted you to them in the first place? Is the relationship worth fighting for, or has your partner turned into someone you feel apart from in too many ways? Every situation is different and there is no one true solution but if you keep love and understanding in your heart you will be on the way to finding the best solution for you.

If you are struggling with caring for your children, perhaps an unruly teenager or a child with behavioural difficulties, this can be one of the most taxing problems ever and cause tremendous strain for all members of the family. Extreme patience is required and you will need more advice than I can give you here, but the one thing I would say is that you hold on to the love you feel for that child. You may not like their behaviour, but you will always love them. Tell them that, and tell them often. It will help you and will help them. If you know you are loved, the world is always a better place whatever is going on in your life.

Looking at the Past – Having Regrets
'It's no use going back to yesterday, because I was a different person then.'
Lewis Carroll, Alice in Wonderland.

As I mentioned earlier, problems from our past are responsible for a lot of the anxieties we suffer from now. Reminders of unhappy memories from the past can come from all manner of things. Perhaps a familiar perfume floating on the air, or a few bars of half-remembered music from long ago is enough to have you catapulted back to a situation you would prefer to forget. At times like this it's a good idea to stop and remind yourself that those days are in the past and although you may wish you could erase them, you can't. You cannot change them either. You may not realise it, but you can learn from those painful memories, even just by becoming a more understanding and empathetic person to others. Ask yourself if the memories are genuinely as bad as you feel they are. Can you try to look back and view them as an outsider and make an objective judgement? If you know it was something completely traumatic, have you ever talked it through with anyone? Until you release the pain and trauma you felt you may have difficulty moving on. Consider talking to a counsellor if this is the case. If you were badly hurt or abused in some way, remember that none of that was your fault. None. You didn't deserve to be treated badly; you deserve to be loved. I don't think many of us can totally stop ourselves from delving into the past in darker moments. We may say to ourselves: 'If this hadn't happened I wouldn't be feeling like this now' or 'if I had acted differently/ taken the job/ moved here instead of there, none of this would have happened and my life would be better.' But how do you know that for sure? We can all find situations and people to blame for how we feel now. Perhaps there is someone to blame or someone who treated you unfairly but that doesn't bring a solution. The solution lies in forgiveness and moving on. Once you have looked at a problem and worked through it then the time will come to stop shining a light on it and to let it fade into insignificance. You are a different person now and what happened, or whatever choices you made in the past are just that. In the past. But you are here now and have a chance to move forward and be who you wish to be. No one can hurt you if you don't let them but you hurt yourself if you cannot let go of past grievances. Buddha says: 'Holding on to anger is like drinking poison and expecting the other person to die'. There is hardly a person on earth who doesn't have some sort of mental scars from the past and maybe that is where a lot of the problems in our world stem from. If we can't show forgiveness and love, to our brothers and sisters at home and all around the world, then troubles occur and escalate. No one is perfect and our upbringing came from those who were doing the best they could from what they themselves had learned along the way.

Getting Older

Getting older is a real fear for a lot of people. When I was doing some research for this book I noticed an interesting pattern emerge. Most of the articles written about the ageing process and the anxiety it provokes seemed to be written by people in their twenties and thirties. At this time of life there is so much peer pressure, and a perception that there is only so much time to achieve all that one aspires to. When juggling a career and trying to raise a family there is much to think about and sometimes there is the worrying thought that time is passing by too quickly. Thoughts about getting wrinkles or experiencing hair loss can both be caused by stress and indeed add to it. Middle age brings new challenges: children become teenagers and leave home to start careers of their own and it is easy for parents to lose direction for a while and feel overwhelmed with emotional turmoil; mothers particularly have the feeling of being made 'redundant'. Thinking positively helps us cope with things like 'empty nest syndrome'; if we can regard it as a new beginning and a time of freedom to take a different path then we will be able to look forward.

People who were well into their prime, i.e., the 'baby boomers', still voiced concerns about ageing at times but were much more able to keep it in perspective and view the passing of time with more of a humorous air. I think this shows us that if we are lucky to go through life and get by relatively unscathed, then we become more content and look both back down the years, and also ahead, with a more philosophical outlook. With age comes wisdom and a way of coping with what may lie ahead. Of course, if we are lucky to stay in good health and keep our mobility and our brains active, this helps us to lead a good and productive life well into our senior years, but for those with health issues then all sorts of problems can worry us. Old age can be more than challenging, and at these times the support of friends, a loving family and caring practitioners can alleviate some of the anxiety that many people face. Sadly, some people do face old age alone and it is, in a way, up to all of us to act with kindness towards others and support and help our neighbours.

Less Obvious Triggers

A lot of the causes of anxiety occur in everyday life, like those mentioned above, and these are easier to recognise than some which aren't visible or obvious. Less obvious things can trigger anxiety even if you are not aware they are is the cause. A few examples of these are:

Being unprepared for what is ahead – i.e. being late for an appointment.

Living in an untidy house.

A low-grade infection.

Oversleeping.

An unexpected bill.

The list is endless…

Who knows what or who can come along to try and spoil our day!

Without becoming too serious, (as that can trigger

anxiety too), it is a good idea to set yourself some tasks which will, in the long-term, help you feel better. Take a good look around at your life and your surroundings. Ask yourself what you are happy with and what could be improved. If you see muddle all around you, develop a system and set about making some small changes; if tidiness is a problem, start by sorting out one room at a time, or even one corner of a room. Once you can see an improvement, however small, you will feel uplifted.

Whilst you are taking a look at your life, ask yourself honestly if you are doing the best you can to keep yourself well. Is it time you had a medical check-up? Do you keep yourself hydrated? So often I realise I have gone through a whole day drinking hardly any water. Dehydration can affect you quite subtly; you may not notice your skin is dry or you are looking a bit peaky and feeling slightly irritable. It may be less beneficial to stop for a cup of tea or coffee than to simply pour a glass of water, but if you can't resist a mid-morning coffee, why not follow it up with a good glug of water? Do this a few times a day and you should notice a gradual difference with your skin and clarity of mind. Even better, fill a large jug with water in the morning and make sure it is empty by the end of the day.

If you find yourself constantly late for work or you regularly oversleep, get into the habit of setting an alarm and getting up half an hour or so earlier than usual. No matter what you have planned for the day, if you start off in a peaceful frame of mind, it will help get you off to a good start. Find a good routine that eases you into the day. Who needs a shrill alarm? That doesn't make sense at all. I have an alarm setting on my mobile phone that wakes me up with a soft gentle melody. (I keep it well away from my pillow but near enough to hear.)

If you find yourself landed with an unexpected bill or something nasty like a parking fine, it is far from ideal. However, it happens and rather than get upset and take things personally (as some of us have been known to with parking fines!) try and keep it in perspective.

So many things can happen and bother us in the course of an average day. Ever heard the expression 'did you get out of the wrong side of the bed?' Of course you have. Some days all sorts of problems can occur but usually they are relatively minor and can be overcome when we remind ourselves that we will have forgotten about them by the end of the week. And even if we haven't, we can work things out. Anger can boil up over something trivial when you are tired or anxious, but if you step back and take a breath you can diffuse a situation. It's not worth falling out with someone or getting upset about something they have said or done. It is not your problem if someone is behaving badly; it is theirs.

The Person You Would Like to Be

I read a quote recently about strong women. It said something like 'Be the person now that you would have liked by your side when you were a child'. Wow. Isn't that something? It stopped me in my tracks. I have been thinking about it ever since.

Do you remember times when, no matter how loving your upbringing, you felt as though no one understood you? Maybe, like me, you were crushed by shyness and wanted to disappear into a hole when someone spoke to you? Or you didn't feel you had anything clever to say. Or you weren't 'with it'? How many times in life have we all encountered difficult situations when a smile or an encouraging word could have made all the difference? Even when perhaps our actions may have been foolish, think how much it would have helped if someone had said, 'Okay, you messed up, but learn from it and move on. I know you are a good person.'

Encouragement is so important. So is understanding and empathy. I see that now, and I yearned for it when I was younger - at school, and later, as a student nurse. And kindness. Kindness is the most important quality in life, I think. A simple act of kindness makes life so much more bearable when times are rough. I know we all have to learn to stand on our own two feet. But how much stronger we feel with someone to fight our corner.

Life is a learning process. Indeed, I am still learning every day; I think I may have been a slow learner. Sometimes I think I may just be getting there and then something happens to take me, temporarily, back to square one. Of course, I am completely grown up now, really quite senior in fact! But there can still be times when I feel like the shy girl in the corner; it's a habit that can stay with you through life if you aren't careful. But I carry on regardless, safe in the knowledge that I am doing my best. One thing is for sure, most of us have small trembles from time to time, whatever our age, but whatever our age, we can gain comfort from the support of our friends.

I am working, still, on being the person I would like to have had at my side all those years ago.

I Wish I'd Known You

I wish I'd known you then
When I couldn't find my voice
When I had no way of knowing
That there could be a choice.
And I wish I'd known you then
When the spotlight fell on me;
A nervous child who didn't know
Who she could one day be.
I wish I'd know you when
I wasn't part of the crowd,
You would have been the one
To call my name out loud.
I wish I'd known you would have
Seen my point of view,
And told me it would be okay
And I'd grow up to be you.

As I mentioned above, when we are in our twenties and thirties we work hard and try hard to fit in. We go through the 'warrior' stage where we feel under pressure to provide for our families and these are the times anxiety can come to the fore.

Striving to be the Best

I have read so much recently about striving. Striving to be the best you can be and striving to find the best life you can have. Instructions on how to manifest what you want and how to order what you want from the universe. This is all fine and interesting and yes, helpful too, but what do you do when you can't keep everything together? Is it sometimes better to focus on the simpler things in life, the small everyday actions that can keep life ticking over? Or is it better to make a start on a new road? Every journey starts with small steps. A big part of the battle against anxiety involves staying in the moment, but also knowing that one day you will move forward. And a big part of that involves staying positive. Keeping focused on the now.

What would make you happy today? This is a good thing to think about. For one thing it stops you thinking about more negative subjects, and another, it can help you take some actions, however small. Ask yourself what small treat you would like, or think about visiting someone you love.

Looking the best you can helps you face the day. Standing up straight and looking confident will make you feel and appear better and automatically warmer and open to others. Think of your aura positively glowing!

How can you create a better atmosphere in your home? Your environment is so important to your mood. Cook simple but wholesome food, light some candles and express gratitude to those who are with you. If you are on your own, make sure you still make the effort. Realise you deserve sympathetic and mellow surroundings.

What do you want to see yourself doing in the future? Picture yourself doing something you have dreamed about. Would you like to look for a different career? Even if you can't think of a way through now, picture it anyway.

When you are in conversation with others, really listen to what they say. Pay them a compliment and make them feel worthwhile. That in turn helps you.

I have made some suggestions here. I haven't gone into too much detail about coping with anxiety as I have given suggestions elsewhere in the book, but I really wanted to focus on ways of letting go. Can we find a way of release; a way to kick up our heels and have a go at feeling good?

What can really help us to both hold on to life and let go of the grip of anxiety?

I was speaking to someone recently who had suffered from anxiety for many years and he explained that for so long fear and worry had stopped him doing so many things. He couldn't hold down a job because there were so many days he couldn't face going to work and called in sick. Eventually those he worked for lost patience. They thought he was lazy and work-shy. They didn't know what really held him back. In all aspects of his life he was afraid and rather than attempt things he gave up at the first hurdle. Then suddenly he realised he had had enough. Enough of just holding on. He finally 'got it'. He decided to let go and see what happened. He saw his friends having fun, leading life to the full and taking risks. He thought to himself he would just go for it, even if he felt anxious. After all, he couldn't really feel any worse than he already did, and at least he would be doing something he could talk about to others. So, he started doing 'normal things'; he travelled, messed around with friends, went on nights out even when he felt bad. The more he did, the more normal he began to feel. Of course, it was important not to overdo it either; late nights and too much alcohol would have been counterproductive here, as would bombarding the senses with too much new activity. But this person was brave enough to meet his anxiety head-on rather than stay in an anxiety cycle.

Another thing to realise is how important talking is. If my friend had talked to his bosses and been honest, he could well have been met with sympathy and understanding - and if not, it would have been good to move on anyway. It takes courage to open up and tell someone you feel bad at times, but you would be surprised how many people will tell you they have been there too. Also, the people who are worth having in your life are the ones who show you compassion and make an effort to understand you. Even if they don't always seem the same as you, if they make an effort and show up, they are worth knowing.

So, by giving yourself a break and having a go at life - putting your worries aside and going through the motions of having a good time - you will save yourself a lot of energy. Have you ever noticed how tiring having an anxious day is?

Have a go at saying to your anxiety 'do what you want - I don't care any more and I am in charge'. You may find that you begin to feel better and the spells of being worry-free become longer.

There are no magic solutions to anything in life and what works for one person will not always work for another. But remember that life is very hard to fathom out at times. For everyone. Momentous times come and go. Some extraordinary, some tragic, some heart-stoppingly beautiful, some you wish you could forget. But the main thing is, if we give it a go, we will look back without regret.

In the words of one of my favourite writers -

'If things start happening, don't worry, don't stew, just go right along and you'll start happening too.'
Dr. Seuss.

Ways of Coping with Anxiety

Just when you think you are doing okay, when you have life worked out at last and have a spring in your step again, do you find yourself 'floored' by a comment you hear in passing or by an unexpected letter stuffed through the letterbox? It may not be anything serious but enough to make you jittery.

Sometimes we can feel we are on a fine balance, and find it hard to cope with extra pressures. Or maybe we don't like the world to see us looking anxious or worried, and so we bottle things up inside. This is worse than letting go and having a meltdown; emotional turmoil can be damaging to us if not released.

I read this explanation of anxiety somewhere and it really resonated with me:

'Anxiety is not being able to sleep because you said something wrong two years ago and can't stop thinking about it.'

This may or may not be true for you, but I know I have had times when I've lain awake tossing and turning, worrying about past mistakes. Maybe, mistakes is not the right word; perhaps it is 'perceived' mistakes. Those things which may not have even been important at the time and certainly aren't now. Then there are the worries that creep in about tomorrow, next week or next year. The 'what ifs' and the 'how is that?' Before I know it an hour or two has passed and then I start fretting about the fact that I can't sleep and worry about being a wreck the next day. Thinking 'I must get to sleep' doesn't help!

The good news is there are things that can help:

Repeat your worries over and over rather than try to push them to the back of your mind. Instead, rumble them around until you are bored with them. It may not be a cure exactly but it is better than being overwhelmed.

Think of the worst thing that could happen in a situation you are worrying about, for example, forgetting what to say when giving a speech. Imagine making light of it and joking with your audience - see yourself relaxing and letting the words flow - people usually understand, they've often been there themselves.

Don't judge yourself if you are feeling a bit 'crazy'. You may think a little strangely at times, but that doesn't mean you are going to act upon your thoughts. Realise that no one is 'normal' and what is normal anyway?

Remember that most things you fear do not come true. If and when they do, then that is the time to take action. Not now. Those panicky feelings are not going to kill you or give you a heart attack, but if you can deflect them by telling yourself most things you are worrying about won't happen you are saving yourself some angst.

Be a casual observer. View your worries from afar and make light of them. See them drift off into the distance and wave them goodbye.

Realise you can't take control of everything. If you feel you've done or said something tactless or silly (most people probably haven't even noticed) don't fret about it. Just be warm and friendly, and smile.

Breathe deeply and slowly when you are anxious - I know you have probably heard this many times before, but it does help. If nothing else, it slows you down and calms the nerves.

Don't let anxiety take over and stop you enjoying things. Even if you think you have a major worry, divide your time – set aside some going-out time to spend an uplifting hour or two with a friend, and then go back to the worry when you get home. Chances are it won't seem nearly so bad.

Most of all, whatever is happening in your life, remind yourself - this too will pass. Nothing lasts forever in life whether good or bad, whoever and wherever you are in life. That is a fact.

What can you still do in life when you are anxious? Actually, almost everything!

Be gentle with yourself. You are doing the best you can.

Coping and Being Loved.

There are many ways of coping with anxiety and different ones work for different people. One thing I have noticed is that friends and family often want to find a solution for you and a reason for why this is happening to you. That's fine but there are times you don't want to listen to solutions and you don't particularly want to have the reasons described. You just want to get through the day. And all you really want is for someone to say: 'It's okay' or 'you will get through this' and 'I am here for you. I love you'. With empathy and support you can cope so much better. Remember - just because a condition is given a label it doesn't necessarily mean it solves the problem in your head.

Here are some tips about what not to do when you are battling with anxiety:

𝔅 *Do not watch the news.*

𝔅 *If you are worried about your health, do not under any circumstances look up the condition you are worried you have on the internet. I promise you the information you find will scare you and often the stuff you read is not accurate. Trust me on this. I have been there!*

𝔅 *Don't overdose on caffeine and be careful with alcohol consumption - hangovers are debilitating at the best of times, but if you are feeling vulnerable they can make anxiety levels worse.*

𝔅 *Do not become a couch potato - you will feel much better if you go outside and walk/take exercise.*

𝔅 *Don't have very late nights. Lack of sleep makes anxiety worse. Even if you suffer from insomnia - get to bed early and get as much sleep as you can. At the same time, rather than lie tossing and turning, get up for a while and make a milky drink (cow's milk, or an alternative such as almond milk, if you don't like dairy). Then try and get back to sleep again.*

❦ *Don't eat junk and sugary foods. Avoid any foods that trigger your anxiety and cause headaches, like cheese and yeast extract, for example. Acid-producing food and drinks can make you jittery i.e. processed meats and sodas, whilst alkaline foods can be more calming, i.e. vegetables and most fruits, beans and lentils.*

If you are trying to help someone with anxiety, here are a few things to remember:

❦ *Often someone in an anxious state comes across as distant or uncaring but this is not how they are inside - they are feeling bad and preoccupied and may not realise how they appear to others. It doesn't mean they don't love or care about you.*

❦ *Don't say their worries are silly or unfounded. They are very real to them!*

❧ *They may appreciate your help but not you trying to change them. You cannot know how they are feeling inside.*

❧ *Never say 'pull yourself together!' (I'm sure you wouldn't!) For those suffering from anxiety, getting through the day is the important thing.*

❧ *When you are in a situation that is causing you to feel anxious - for example, worrying you might be late for an appointment, or losing your keys, ask yourself what would be the worst thing that could happen? Most things can be overcome even if they upset us at the time and cause an inconvenience. You will find most people are helpful if you are stuck in a minor predicament. Try and reach out and have a light-hearted approach - it is amazing how this will help an awkward situation and make you feel more optimistic.*

❧ *Even in more serious situations that would make most people anxious, you will be surprised how you will often find help and sympathy from unexpected people or places.*

❧ *Remember, anxiety doesn't define you.*

❧ *Have a small item that you find comforting and keep it with you. I have a few words on a scrap of paper in my handbag written by my late mother - it reads: 'To my lovely girl - be happy. You will never know how much I love you. Love, Mum.' To know you are loved or have been loved is more than uplifting. It is at the core of everything.*

❧ *YOU are loved. Yes, you are - even if you doubt it.*

Worrying about the World

A nxiety affects so many of us and not least when we worry about the unrest in our world. In recent times we have witnessed the heart-breaking results of terrorism, starvation, war and the resultant effects it has on innocent people. Sometimes we feel so dismayed and yet feel helpless. We look on in frustration and wonder why we can't all live side by side in peace.

When we feel worried about the world and can't see an end to all the unrest that worries us, it is good to try and take a step back and look at our beautiful world from afar. I am not saying there is an instant solution, but it helps put things into perspective. Imagine yourself looking down at our world from a space-ship. What do you see? Do you see lines and labels or huge dividing walls? Do you see any big names written across the landscape? No. You just see rugged landscape and large expanses of water. That's it. The maps we have been taught to use are useful of course – we need to know our way around and find our bearings in the world, but maps are just pieces of paper with reference points and made-up names used to help human travelling. Once we realise this, we see there are no real separations, only man-made barriers, and it is just the same with our minds and thinking – the barriers we put up are not real but imagined. So if we can think differently we will be well on the way to viewing ourselves and the world with fresh eyes.

Coping with Difficult Days

It is hard not to think about heartbreak and sadness - so much has happened in our world to render us bereft and fearful. Our hearts are troubled as more and more tragic, dreadful and appalling occurrences unfold in front of our eyes as we view our television screens. How much can some people take, we ask ourselves; what can we do to help others and also keep ourselves safe? We become full of doubt - how can this happen? Why are people around the world suffering in such awful ways? There may be some who in their hearts know the answers, but for most of us we have to carry on somehow, and meanwhile the books of condolences are filled with words from grieving hearts, and the flowers continue to be laid all around the sites of the latest disaster.

At times we do not wake refreshed and we find it hard to concentrate on our daily routine. I think that any extreme is hard to cope with. We search for equilibrium and balance in all things - at least I do. It's easier to cope with life when we can jog along at a steady pace, walk around without feeling fearful of what lurks around the corner, and know that everything is in order. But of course, nothing stays like that for long, and when things go badly wrong we have to dig deep to find strength to cope. It is at times like these that the smallest things seem to help us - getting out into the garden, walking in the woods, hugging the grandchildren and reading them a funny story. We can share a coffee with friends, help our neighbour, and offer someone a word or two of kindness. Just going through the motions of routine tasks can get us through the days that are difficult.

As always in times of dreadful disaster, we see the kindness of strangers shine through. People pull together and are incredibly brave and courageous. They give. They give money they don't really have; they give people comfort, both materially and physically; they give love and show compassion. That's when we realise how much goodness there is in this time of utmost suffering.

We often find that the wider our experience is, the deeper our tolerance. Wisdom comes from all the ups and downs we have gone through in our lives and how we have dealt with them. And with wisdom comes a knowing. Knowing not to give advice unless asked for it; not making assumptions and forming opinions; not making judgements. It's knowing we don't always get things right and being ready to hold our hands up and admit it when we get things wrong. Mainly wisdom gives us courage. Courage to reach out when we see someone in need even if we have to step out of our comfort zone to help them. Courage to face our own demons. Courage to step out and keep going in this scary world. Courage to stand up for what we believe in a peaceful, honest and informed manner.

One of my sons once said to me that it is what we do when no one is looking that counts, and I have found this to be so true in life. If we can go forth with a light heart, we can find it easier to cope with that which life throws at us.

In these times of darkness, we pray for all those whose

hearts are breaking. We pray they will find some peace and will be wrapped in the love and comfort of open and loving arms.

Most of all we remember that when we all look to the future with love in our hearts, and unite in peace, we will be lifted up together.

The Diary of a Life

I remember a little girl of about six or seven attending her art lesson at school. She loved art and painting and being creative. She had looked forward to her lesson for a full week; she had planned the picture she wanted to paint in her mind, and went excitedly in to the art room. She loved the smell of the paint and the rather chaotic aspect of the airy room with its old, paint-splattered benches and the canvases stacked against the wall. This was a place where, for a while, she could get a bit messy and nobody minded. She put on her apron and collected together some paintbrushes and paint and placed them on the table in front of her. She laid down some paper and sketched an outline of the scene she wanted to paint. Lost in her own world, she spent her time lovingly drawing the picture. Her teacher looked over her shoulder from time to time and made encouraging noises. She mixed her paints and carefully started painting. Her picture began to come alive and she was sure this was going to be her best work yet. She looked at the pretty rural scene, its sunny blue sky and birds and butterflies, and was happy. The other classmates looked at her work with admiring glances. She couldn't wait to pin her work on the wall. She pushed back her chair quickly, ready to take her picture to the teacher. In her haste, her elbow knocked over her pot of dirty paint water, and, rooted to the spot, she watched as the water seeped across the paper in front of her. All the colours ran into one another, mixing together and fanning out in all directions until the picture beneath was indistinguishable. There was silence in the class. Tears welled up in the little girl's eyes and dropped on to the picture. But the little girl's teacher smiled. 'You had painted a very pretty picture,' she said, 'but I think this one will be a lot more special. Look how the colours are flowing into one another and creating something beautiful to look at. There are shapes and swirls which will help the viewer to use their imagination when they look at it. It would grace any wall. So don't be sad.' As the painting dried it did indeed look beautiful and the little girl dried her tears. The teacher framed the picture and pinned it on the wall in the art room as an example of abstract art. At the end of term, the little girl was awarded the art prize for her year.

The above is just one small example of how an unexpected occurrence can change our path or our viewpoint. At a young age, a lesson that teaches us to view a potential disaster with equanimity is a good thing, but so many times life throws us a curve ball and we flounder – 'But I had planned to do this or that,' we say; 'I don't want to downsize because my finances dictate it!' or 'I haven't got time to be ill!' How do we cope when life changes unexpectedly? It's not easy. As the quote by Allen Saunders goes – 'Life is what happens to us while we are making other plans.'

It may be hard at times to adjust, and of course some life changes are much harder to cope with than others. I ask myself now if I would go back to the house I loved and left six years ago. It was traumatic at the time for various reasons, but now I have a different life; I live in different surroundings and have downsized considerably. I enjoy the environment I now live in and enjoy spending time with new people I have met. It's not what I would have chosen, but it's good. With the love of good friends and family, we can cope with change.

For those coping with illness it is harder still. For those

facing illness or surgery, life can alter unimaginably. I think then, especially, it's clinging on to the small things that can help. Trying to keep to a routine so that life still seems relatively normal seems to help. Often I read of someone who has faced illness and has come through the other side, and they are grateful. Grateful in some way for having been ill as it had enabled them to take stock and to look at life in a different way. That, to me, is bravery.

'The life of every man is a diary in which he means to write one story, and writes another; and his humblest hour is when he compares the volume as it is with what he vowed to make it.'
J.M.Barrie The Little Minister

Diversion Tactics

There are several ways we can help ourselves cope with anxiety and once you become proactive in aiding your recovery you will start to feel more positive. It's just taking these first steps that is the hardest! As it is said – every journey has to start with a single step. Why not try a few things and find out what works best for you?

Mindfulness and Meditation

Paying more attention to the present moment – to your own thoughts and feelings, and to the world around you can improve your mental well-being. Some people call this awareness 'mindfulness'. Mindfulness can help us enjoy life more and understand our own life better.

As we all know, it is easy when feeling low to want to hide away from the world. This makes us stop noticing what is going on around us and before we know it we lose touch with the way our bodies are feeling and end up totally caught up in our own thoughts. We forget what drives our emotions and behaviour. Mindfulness helps us reconnect with our bodies and normal sensations. It may sound so simple. But even waking up our senses by walking round with bare feet and feeling the grass beneath our feet or the wind in our hair can help us feel more connected to life. Once we learn to live in the moment again we can be more aware of our thoughts as they happen and thus view life more clearly and positively. We may also see what we may have been taking for granted. Mindfulness also lets us see where our negative thoughts have been taking us and what normally triggers them. If we stand back from our thoughts and see their patterns we can learn which patterns of thinking to avoid. We can see that mental events do not have to control us. When we start to get introspective we can ask ourselves why we are thinking this way and if we are just getting caught up in our thoughts.

I for one know that even with all the best intentions, it is not easy to step away from worries and unhappy thoughts. A good way of dealing with this is to admit that negative thoughts are 'events' that can be put to one side. Imagine standing by a stream and seeing some rafts floating by with your thoughts on board. You don't have to get on the raft with the thoughts; you can let them drift off without you. It may take a while to get used to doing this but it will get easier with practice.

Meditation

Meditation is again about quietening and resting the mind and is especially helpful in controlling unwanted thinking. You can start off with just a few minutes each day, sitting quietly and comfortably and finding an inner state in your mind where you can be silent and no longer distracted by events going on around you. I find meditating quite hard to do and I don't set any rules or become too involved in complicated chanting, although finding a simple mantra (a word you can repeat over and over again to help you find calm and focus) that you like is very soothing. There are many mantras you can choose, perhaps from a number of Sanskrit (ancient and sacred) mantras which have meaning in the words and sounds, (just google Sanskrit mantras!) Or you can simply choose one of your own words.

Both meditation and mindfulness have the potential to

improve your ability to cope with anxiety and stress. One of the main reasons is that they both help with your breathing which is one of the issues that makes anxiety feel worse, especially if you unfortunately suffer with scary panic attacks which are often accompanied with uneven and shallow breathing. Most forms of meditation start by concentrating on 'correct breathing technique'. I also believe that the spiritual qualities of meditation helps to cure, or at the very least, help you cope with anxiety. Often people say they haven't the time to put aside for meditation, but actually meditation gives you more time by making your mind calmer and more focused. A simple ten or fifteen-minute breathing meditation can help you find some inner peace and balance. It can also help you to understand your own mind and move from feeling negative to positive and unhappy to happy.

Some people will find it easier to relax their minds with gentle yoga. Yoga is an ancient form of exercise that focuses on strength, flexibility and breathing to boost physical and mental well-being. The main components of yoga are postures and movements to benefit health and flexibility. There are various forms of yoga and some are more vigorous than others, so the key is to find a class appropriate to your fitness levels.

There are many websites dedicated to meditation, mindfulness and yoga and I will list some at the end of the book.

Medication

Most of us do not like to think about taking medication to help alleviate anxiety and depression, which is understandable. Nevertheless, there is nothing to be ashamed of if it is the best option for you and it is certainly something your doctor will want to discuss with you if you are struggling to feel better. There are types of depression which result from a chemical imbalance in the brain and if you think of antidepressant medicine as just a replacement for something you are lacking, you may be more open to giving medication a try. Just keep in mind they can take a while to build up in the body and take effect, so it is best to give them a fair trial. Sometimes, combining a course of medication with the above suggestions such as exercise and meditation may be a really good solution in helping you move forward.

There are several herbal remedies available for helping

with mild anxiety which can be useful. They are said to provide mild sedation without side effects, but I would recommend that you talk to a health practitioner or pharmacist before taking them as some can interact with prescribed drugs. St John's wort and valerian are two well-known herbs which are used for mild anxiety with reportedly good results; but again, please check first that they are suitable for you.

Essential Oils

Essential oils can have a very powerful effect on our mood, emotions and behaviour. For anxiety, essential oils such as bergamot, basil, clary sage, frankincense, lavender and ylang-ylang have been shown to be helpful. One of the most effective uses for essential oils is in treating anxiety. Aromatherapy massage is very relaxing and enjoyable and if it helps relieve anxiety as well, what could be better?

If you want to enjoy essential oils at home, it is good to have a diffuser or burner and create your own uplifting blends to fragrance the air and lift the spirits.

Through the Eyes of a Child

I have watched several children's television programmes with my grandchildren and recently, whilst watching with one of them, I realised how differently we see the world when looking through the eyes of a child. This may sound so obvious, but it is worth thinking about.

Notice how much brighter the colours are in our children's favourite story. See too, how good prevails, magic is commonplace and anything can happen! Laughter comes easily, and, rain or shine, the everyday world is fun. Problems are usually worked around and overcome. It is sad to think that as we get older we worry more about what people think and even become cynical.

Life is far from perfect, and sometimes bad things happen to good people, but if we can stop and look at the colours, believe in a bit of magic, and take time to jump in a few puddles then maybe we will walk with a bit of a spring in our step. Maybe we can all grow a bit by looking through the eyes of a child.

Life tends to be about rushing forward and waiting for the next event in our lives, but if we can stop from time to time and embrace childish things we will feel the benefit.

'If you want your child to be intelligent, read them fairy tales. If you want them to be more intelligent, read them more fairy tales'.

Albert Einstein

'The Moving Finger writes; and having writ,
Moves on: nor all thy Piety nor Wit,
Shall lure it back to cancel half a Line,
Nor all thy Tears wash out a Word of it'.

Omar Khayyam (1048? – 1122)
Omar Khayyam was a scholar and astronomer who lived in Iran. His poetry reflects his thoughts about life and this quote has not diminished in the passing of time.

Giving, Receiving and Finding Courage

Have you ever noticed how much easier it is to give than receive? Of course, it is wonderful to give a gift, whether it is a material gift or the gift of your time, friendship, love or support. To see someone's face light up with the pleasure of receiving a gift you have chosen or to know you have helped someone, perhaps during a crisis, makes both you as well as the recipient feel good, or at least better, depending on the gift and the circumstances. But during bouts of anxiety there are times when we can feel unworthy and find it hard to accept help when it is offered. Maybe we feel that we don't matter, and we are in a place where we find it hard to see the value in what is being offered, or perhaps we don't even have the necessary energy to take new opportunities that are laid in front of us.

When it is hard to receive love for fear of the consequences of letting down your defences, it might be that you are trying to remain emotionally strong so that you don't have to face possible hurts that letting yourself love might bring. But it is important to be able to receive love so that you can feel like a whole person and have a real sense of self-worth. It is important to be able to trust someone when they say they love you and take it at face value. It is easy to start questioning their gift of love and be afraid they do not mean it. This may result in you turning someone away and missing out on an important part of your life.

Again it is easy for the old fears about loss to creep in. If previous relationships have ended due to death or break-up or because of an episode from the past that has scarred you, you may be unwilling to put yourself out there again and open up to the possibility of being happy. But if you embrace new love that is willingly offered, go with the flow, and have good expectations, the chances are that life could change for the better. Once you open your heart and live in the moment and realise that others care about you, you will feel needed and wanted. This is a great feeling and can set you on the path to feeling better about yourself and being in a good place mentally.

Beware of social negativity. Social conditioning has the habit of making us feel wary of giving and receiving compliments. You may feel you are attracting too much of the limelight, but when someone pays you a lovely compliment, smile and give thanks!

We can think of how children give and receive love. They don't worry about how and when they should give and receive love – they just say what they feel with complete honesty and spontaneity. And they ask for help when they need it!

We often tell children to stop behaving like a child and grow up…yet when we tap into our inner child and embrace childlike wonder, we can improve our lives.

'Keep the love you have been given in your heart. It will stay with you long after all the other gifts of life have vanished.'

Courage

Courage takes many forms. Wikipedia explains it thus: 'Courage is the choice and willingness to confront agony, pain, danger, uncertainty or intimidation. Physical courage is bravery in the face of physical pain, hardship, death or threat of death, while moral courage is the ability to act rightly in the face of popular opposition, shame, scandal, discouragement or personal loss.'

The above passage explains courage very well. But here I want to write about the sort of courage you have to find deep inside you when facing up to your fears. There is no point in comparing fears and the different ways we face them and no way of differentiating between what are big fears and what are small ones. If you are fearful about something then it is a big fear to you. To me, the main quality that makes someone courageous is when they act with fortitude. If you can find the will to go out there and face those difficulties you have and diffuse them with your inner strength, then you are indeed courageous. Having such a quality doesn't come easily as we are often scared of those very difficulties. Remind yourself that no one is fearless. The people we admire that act courageously are actually the ones who have found a way of moving through their fear. That is exciting for us as it shows that it is more than possible to rise above our fears; with practice, debilitating fears can be overcome.

If we try and forget about everything that surrounds our fear and we get rid of all the drama we feel could come from a bad outcome, we can be more logical and tell ourselves we are just having the same feelings that all human beings have, and we are actually on the verge of growth! Being brave means taking steps in spite of being fearful. Whatever is worrying you, put it into words, perhaps with a trusted friend or counsellor or even in your prayers! Just voicing your fears can be enough to take you on a path to recovery or solution.

Another thing to remember is that focusing on another person's problem not only can help them but can put your own worries into perspective. Because with courage comes kindness; kindness matters, and it is one of the greatest attributes you can have and show to others.

Being courageous isn't easy at times. But if you step outside of you comfort zone and put your best foot forward you can feel better.

> *'Life is mostly froth and bubble,*
> *Two things stand in stone.*
> *Kindness in another's trouble,*
> *Courage in your own.'*

Adam Lindsay Gordon

'My religion is very simple. My religion is kindness.'

Dalai Lama

'Promise me you'll always remember:
You're braver than you believe, and stronger than you seem,
and smarter than you think.'

A.A. Milne

How Do You Move Forward?

I have written about anxiety and how it can affect us in so many ways - from the way we sound and appear, to how we can be affected physically. Even when we deal well with anxiety, the anxious thoughts still sometimes hover and wait in the wings - waiting for the guard to drop and the mindfulness to lose its helpful grip for a while. If, like me, you spend a lot of time reading about self-help and enlightenment you will know what I mean when I say that mindfulness and reaching that absolute place of understanding where we 'get it' and nothing can bother us any more is definitely an ongoing process which needs constant monitoring! (Although, if you have 'got it' you may well disagree with me…actually, you probably won't be reading this anyway, you will be somewhere on cloud nine.)

I can't recall a time in the past when there was so much

helpful information readily available to us on the subject of self-help and spiritual fitness. It's a good thing. It's a great and empowering thing. There is something for all of us, whether we lean towards religious solace, a healthier body and mind, spiritual advancement, meditation, yoga, finding the best retreat, positivity workshops…I could go on…

The benefit in all this help and information is huge. With all the help at our disposal we will find something beneficial for us for sure. We will, sooner or later, have our own particular author or life-style guru who really speaks to us and shows us a way forward when we need it.

I was a nurse for many years, and I can think of countless times when I had to dig deep and give comfort. To be able to reach out and support people in times of tremendous need was of utmost importance, especially when busy and working in a stressful environment. I hope I gave my best. Mostly I feel I did. But it would have been good to have had more helpful ways of releasing the tension after a busy shift than going to the pub around the corner from the hospital! Maybe I wasn't ready then to read the books that would have been helpful - perhaps I was finding my own way then and gaining experience in life. It is said that the teacher comes when the pupil is ready.

And I think it is good to remind ourselves sometimes that simple acts of kindness are within us all. To remember that inherent wisdom and compassion is deep within us, and is even embedded in our DNA. We are braver and wiser than we think. Mindfulness and deep thinking has been around far longer than we have. Self-help is not really new. Ancient philosophers had figured out life over 2,000 years ago. Quotes from so long ago never cease to amaze me and make me realise that everything changes yet nothing changes!

'No man ever steps in the same river twice, for it's not the same river and he's not the same man.'
Heraclitus (lived around 500 years BC in Ephesus.)

Like many big thinkers, Heraclitus was born wealthy in a city, but lived in the woods to contemplate the universe.

'The sage is ready to use all situations and doesn't waste anything. This is called embodying the light.'
Lao Tzu alive around 600 BC in China.

Lao Tzu started Taoism 2,500 years ago in China. He was

legendary - Lao Tzu really just means 'old man' and nobody knows who he actually was. He certainly made a big impression! More importantly, he left us the 'Tao Te Ching' which is full of ancient wisdom.

'To rank the effort above the prize may be called love.'
Confucius (alive in China around 500 BC.)

Confucius is probably the most influential person in Chinese history. He emphasised what we today call grit: finding the value in trying and not just arriving.

'The unexamined life is not worth living.'
Socrates (lived in Athens around 450 BC.)

Socrates embodied the fundamental spirit of Western thought, that you have the responsibility of being in charge of your own life.

Perhaps the most beautiful words of all:

'Out beyond ideas of wrongdoing and rightdoing there is a

field. I'll meet you there. When the soul lies down in that grass
the world is too full to talk about.'

Rumi (poet, born 1207.)

So, today we are lucky with the resources we have - both the old and the new. We may just need to remind ourselves to open our hearts to new learning. To rid ourselves of negative thoughts and change our thinking so we can move forward with positivity and embrace change whilst learning from the past. Nothing, and I mean nothing that is good, is ever lost even when it is centuries old.

As human beings we will always be searching for a newer, better and easier way to find fulfilment. Next time your heart is a little heavy, just remember there is always a way forward. And, as I have said before, if you are anxious you are not alone. You can take comfort from the fact that for centuries we have yearned to find new wisdom and ways to help us move forward and probably will for centuries to come. And we have survived.

Walk the Glittery Path - an excerpt from 'Notes from Dove Lane'.

As we wound our way around the village and walked back up the hill towards the woods behind Dove Lane, the path beneath our feet sparkled in the sun. Looking more closely, I could see there were hundreds of glass chips embedded in the tarmac. I had never noticed this before; maybe it was the direction of the sun or the time of day, but the effect was magical. The path glittered like something out of a fairy tale and I half expected to be transported to a different land. I thought about the beauty that surrounds us, whoever we are and whatever our circumstances; rich or poor, we are all entitled to walk along a glittery pathway.

We are all created as equals. Sometimes it is easy to forget that. I certainly do. I think most of us, at some time in our lives, have looked up at someone we see as more famous, wealthy or seemingly more accomplished than ourselves and felt a little overshadowed. It is a habit that is hard to shake off. But we all have our skills, our own uniqueness that no-one can take away. We can all have a chance to shine and take a walk in the sunshine. There are so many unsung heroes we may pass along the way; those who carry on in the direst circumstances, and still raise a smile.

I sat in the sunshine drinking tea with a friend today and we talked about life; how things sometimes surprise us and turn out differently than expected. How sometimes it's hard to take the rough with the smooth. How busy life can be at times. But would we really want to walk in anyone else's shoes, however important they are?

I love this Malagasy proverb –

'A canoe does not know who is King, when it turns over, everyone gets wet.'

I hope you can walk the glittery path today.

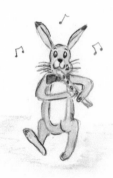

Soothing Music and Helpful Books

So many people have helped me along the way. Here is a list of the ones that really, really are my 'go-to' treasures.

Music

Clifford T. Ward – a singer and songwriter gone from us far too soon and one whose music is forever beautiful, with heartfelt lyrics and melodies. Try the album 'The Ways of Love'.

Any CD by Bliss – 'A Hundred Thousand Angels' which features the wonderful Lucinda Drayton is beautiful.
www.bliss-music.com
www.lucindadrayton.com

'Stillness' – Meditation music from Brahma Kumaris –
www.brahmakumaris.org
(Brahma Kumaris is a worldwide spiritual movement
dedicated to personal transformation and world renewal.)

Track from – The Very Best of Dusty Springfield –
'Goin' Back'.

'Poems, Prayers and Promises' the album – John Denver.

'Secret Garden' – Songs from a Secret Garden.

Cat Stevens – 'Morning Has Broken' from the album
'Teaser and the Firecat'.

Elton John – 'Your Song'. You probably have it!

'What a Wonderful World' – Louis Armstrong.

'Dear Lord and Father of Mankind'- Even if hymns are not
your thing, the words are as profound as they are
everlasting. (Available in any hymnbook!)

Books

Dr Wayne Dyer – Wayne Dyer has written many books. Known as the 'father of motivation', his words have greatly changed my life. To learn more about him and his life go to: www.drwaynedyer.com

Winnie-the-Pooh – A.A. Milne.

The Happiness Project – Gretchen Rubin.

The Alchemist – Paul Coelho.

Better the Whole World Against Me Than My Soul – Wolfgang Sonnenburg

The Color of Water – James McBride – A wonderful book dedicated to mothers.

Helpful and informative websites:

www.mercola.com – Natural Health Information – Articles and health news.

www.oceanrobbins.com – Ocean is passionate about healthy foods which is fair-trade, naturally sustainable and delicious.

www.calmclinic.com

www.mindful.org

www.mind.org.uk

www.headspace.com

UK Health Radio – A health information station with in-depth information on a wide range of health and wellness topics. Also incorporates an online magazine entitled Health Triangle Magazine. www.ukhealthradio.com

There are many yoga websites. If you are looking for a yoga class near you, it's a good idea to enquire at your local library for information.

Acknowledgements

My love and thanks to Brian Halvorsen – I couldn't have got this book (or my life) together without your helpful and loving input.

About Lyn

Lyn Halvorsen is a writer, blogger, and follower of all things inspirational.

Other books by Lyn:

Under the Same Stars – Poems and Illustrations.

Tea at Raphael's – A novel.

Children's Books:

Anton the Brave Viking.

Anton the Brave Viking and the Scaredy Cat.

Anton and the King of Crumbly Castle.

Anton and the Waffle Mountain.

You can read more about Lyn and follow her blog at:

www.notesfromdovelane.com